I give up

by Alan Curson
with illustrations by Fiona Patchett

Published by Alan Curson through Lulu.com
July 1st 2007

Copyright Alan Curson 2007
The moral right of the author has been asserted.

All rights reserved
Without limiting any rights under copyright reserved above, no part of this publication may be reproduced stored in or introduced into a retrieval system, or transmitted in any form or by any means (electronic, mechanical, photocopying, recording or otherwise) without the prior written permission of the copyright owner of this publication.

ISBN 978-0-9556765-0-5

About the author

Alan Curson has worked as an advertising copywriter for more years than he cares to remember. He gave up smoking for good in 1987, using the methods outlined in the following pages, having been a serial "stop-starter" since his teens. The amount of time that has passed since then, while not necessarily a great advertisement for his ability to hit tight deadlines, is a testament to how well the method works. He hasn't touched a single cigarette in that time and more importantly, hasn't wanted to.

Alan Curson lives with his partner Pepita and two children in southwest London.

This really is a short book. Easy to follow, easy to do.

You are just a few quick steps away from becoming a non smoker.

Contents

Introduction
Step one. Prepare yourself
Step two. Commit yourself
Step three. Take action
Step four. Make it work for you
Step five. Picture it
And finally...

I give up

**A step by step guide
to becoming a non smoker**

Thanks to...

Pepita for typing the original draft.
Leon for the chance comment that set me thinking.
Shaun Patchett for his help with design and layout.
Everyone who buys this book.

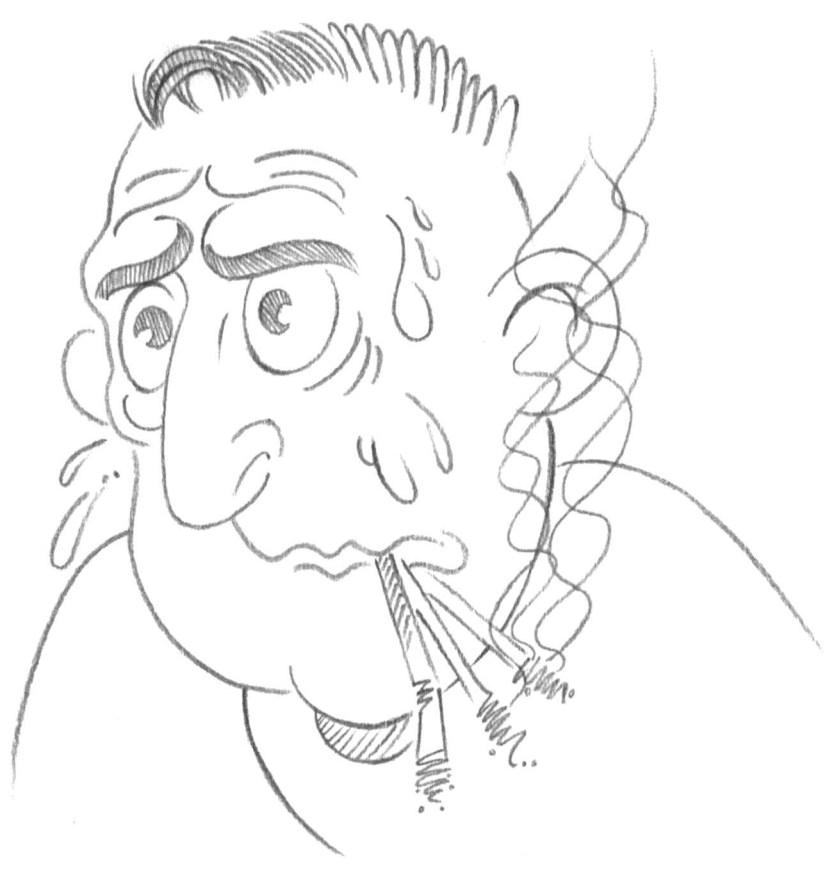

Giving up is easy.
I've done it dozens of times.

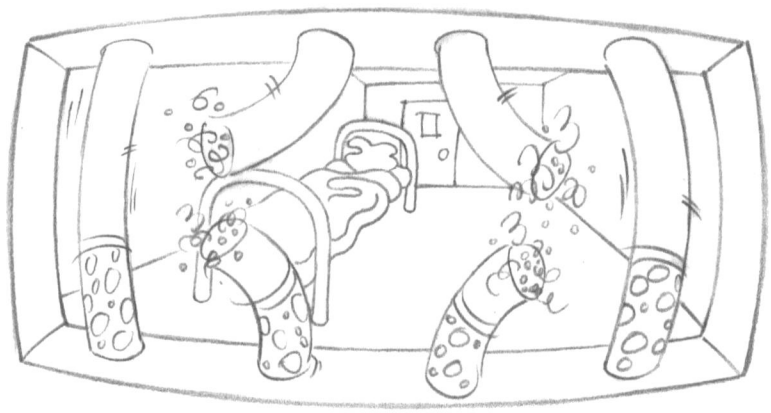

It's time to break out of your nicotine prison

Introduction:

Anything written about giving up smoking has, by definition, to include some suggestions on how to do it. But this isn't just about how to stop. As you'll read, stopping's actually not that hard to do. It's about something much more difficult. Staying stopped.

Anyone who's ever tried to kick the habit, knows the desire to smoke lingers on long (sometimes years) after the last puff. Yet I have read that it takes about 72 hours for the body to withdraw from the chemical addiction to nicotine and the withdrawal symptoms are relatively mild.

So there must be something far more powerful than nicotine keeping us hooked and encouraging us to lapse.

A psychiatrist could probably explain all this in great depth and detail. But for me, the realisation that beating nicotine was only part of the battle was crucial to finally stubbing out the habit for good.

It struck me that the one thing we are all addicted to is our image of ourselves. We are extremely attached to being "us". What makes us "us", are all our little behaviour patterns, habits and mannerisms. And the smaller and more unconscious these mannerisms are, the less we are aware of them.

When we stub out our last cigarette, we also stub out all the little gestures, habits, and micro-behaviours that go with being a smoker. The problem with this is that all these behaviour patterns have been part of us for as long as we've smoked. So when we stop, it can feel like we stop being ourselves.

Most people approach giving up in one of two ways:

1. The "Will power" approach. This involves actively trying to "fight" the urge to smoke.

2. "Evasion" - Zoning out in the hope that the urge will have gone away by the time they zone back in again.

The will power approach creates open warfare between two sections of your own ego. One part hanging on tenaciously to who you are (your behaviours and mannerisms) the other part doing its utmost to change you by force. The second approach essentially involves trying to forget who you are, which your ego won't allow for very long.

At best neither approach offers more than an uneasy truce between the smoking you and the non-smoking you.

I'm not saying you can't give up this way. I'm sure many people have. And in fact, these approaches could be very useful in the initial giving up stage.

However, I think there's a much easier way, one that works with your ego rather than against it.

A way that helps you become a genuine non smoker.

The following pages contain a way of looking at this problem and dealing with it, which helped me change from a 30 a day smoker to a person who doesn't smoke and has no cravings whatsoever to do so. It doesn't take iron will power. It's just a matter of getting into the right mind-set and following a few simple guidelines.

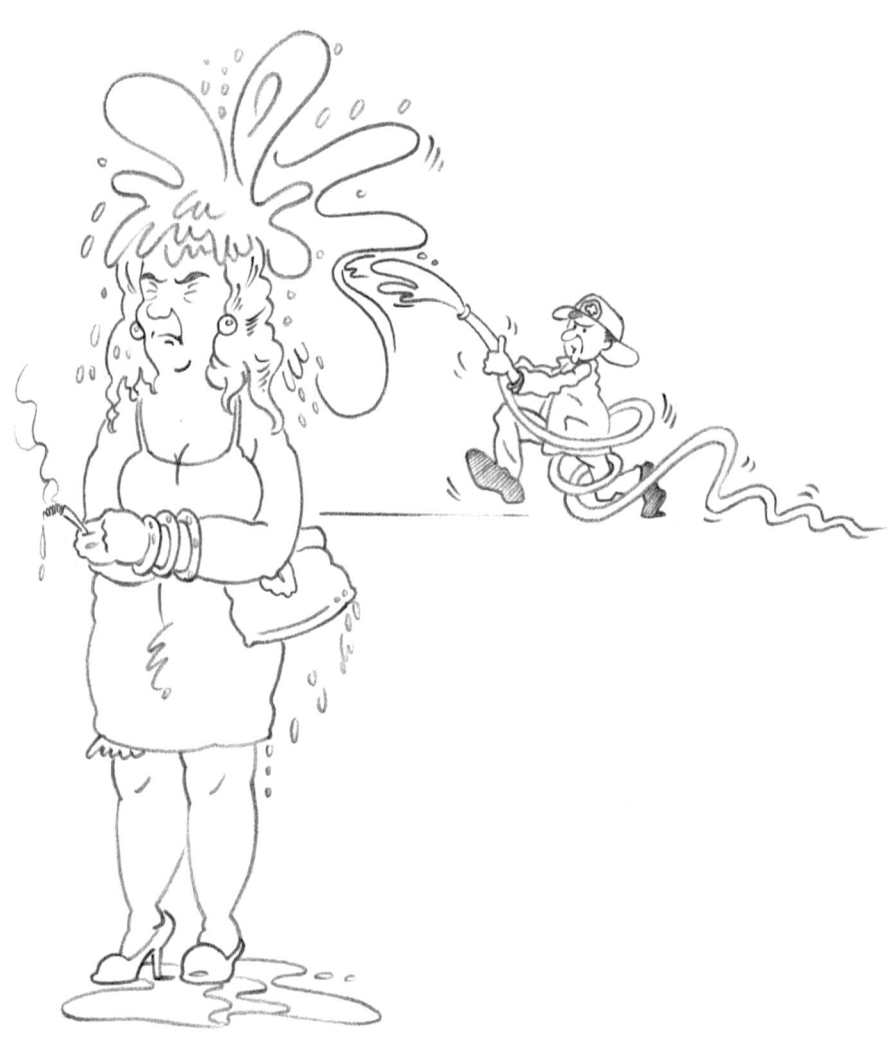

Smoking's a great way to meet nice Firemen

Step 1. Prepare yourself

In case you need a reason why.

☞ *Everyone knows smoking's bad for you. But to help strengthen your resolve and encourage you to "start stopping" today, here are a few of the problems smoking can cause:*

☞ *Smoking damages your lungs, your heart, your eyes, your arteries, your brain, your sex life, your mouth, your throat and practically everything else.*

☞ *Smoking makes you cough.*

☞ *Smoking makes you smell, it makes your clothes smell, it makes your furniture and your home smell.*

- *Smoking makes your car smell.*

- *It even makes your children smell.*

- *Smoking is a pretty effective way of setting fire to things you'd rather not set fire to, including yourself. In fact, fires started by cigarettes kill more people than any other kind of fire.*

- *Ashtrays smell and are ugly. Cigarette ends make horrible litter.*

- *Smoking is an ugly habit to watch.*

- *Smoking stains your fingers yellow.*

- *Smoking destroys your sense of taste and smell.*

- *If you smoke, younger, more impressionable people who look up to you (eg your children), may try to copy you.*

- *Smoking is expensive. A packet a day is equivalent to a trip to the West Indies once a year.*

- *Smoking is the leading cause of blindness in older people and because it causes small blood vessels to fail, it can result in the amputation of legs and arms.*

- *Smoking causes lung cancer, heart disease, throat cancer and many, many other nasty, painful, life threatening conditions.*

☞ *Smoking doesn't just harm you. It harms people around you who are forced to become passive smokers in your presence. (People like your children.)*

☞ *Smoking stains your teeth.*

☞ *Smoking speeds up the ageing of your skin and encourages wrinkles to form.*

☞ *Smoking makes a group of cynical people very rich. Every puff you take breathes profit into the balance books of rich tobacco companies.*

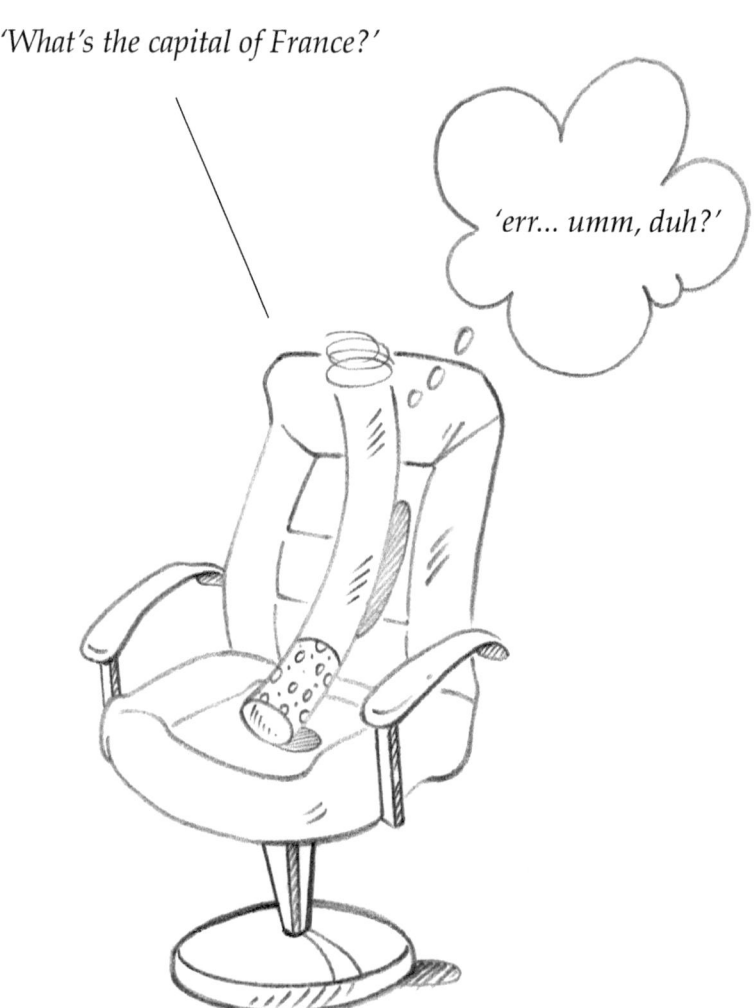

Cigarettes are really stupid

Step 2. Commit yourself

After you've read my list of reasons to stop, write down the ones that you feel might apply to you. Then see if you can think of any other reasons and write these down, too.

I found writing things like this down, helped me to make a clear commitment. It also prevented me from fudging the issue, avoiding it, putting it off or kidding myself into believing it didn't really matter whether I stopped or not.

Once you've written your list, it's hard to avoid the fact that there are no good reasons for smoking and there are hundreds of good reasons for not doing it.

If you think about it, given the down side, you'd have to be barmy to want to carry on smoking.

So while you're still addicted, the first thing is to admit to yourself that you're not smoking because it's a good thing, you're smoking because the addiction makes you want to smoke.

Now, commit yourself. Write down why you think smoking is stupid, then sign it.

I know it's obvious that smoking is a bad thing, but you'd be surprised how much it helps to just write it down. (Remember you aren't even committing yourself to stopping yet. Just to the idea that smoking is a stupid, unpleasant and dangerous habit which doesn't make any sense)

The only question now is not whether you're going to stop, but when you're going to stop.

All I can say about this, is do it when it suits you.

Maybe is will be easier if you choose a time when you know you'll be relaxed, like on holiday. Maybe it will be better for you to choose a time when you are busy and have lots of distractions.

The important thing is to make a decision that feels right

and stick to it.

'I'm giving up"

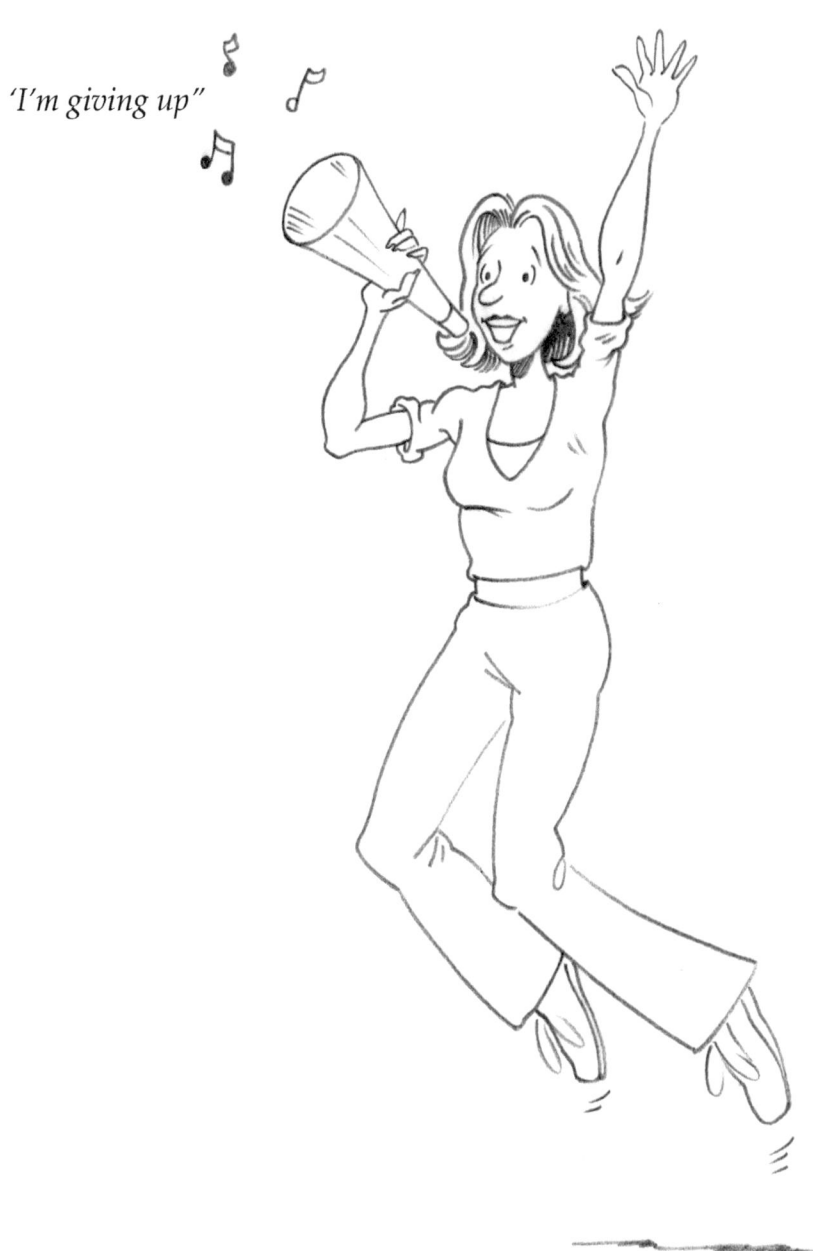

Make a song and dance about it if you want

Don't prevaricate. This is something you just have to go for. And the worse that can happen if you fail (not that you're going to fail if you follow the advice in this little booklet) is that you'll be no worse off than you are right now.

If it helps to make a song and dance about it and tell all your friends what you're doing, go ahead and tell them. If on the other hand, you'd rather just quietly get on and do it, then quietly get on and do it.

But do it.

As you read earlier, stopping's not the hardest part. In fact it's quite easy.

If you don't believe me, think about this. Every night, most smokers sleep for as long as eight hours without a cigarette. With no problems whatsoever. If the addiction was as strong as it seems, it would wake you every hour or so for another fix, wouldn't it. But it doesn't.

Imagine being a smoker and going without for eight hours at a stretch during the day. That would be like, well stopping, really wouldn't it.

The truth is, you give it up every night to go to sleep. So giving it up is something you can and in fact, do every day.

What really counts is staying stopped.

Here are a few approaches that may help you over the first hurdle:

Acupuncture

Don't knock it if you haven't tried it. Some people swear by it and medical research is beginning to show that acupuncture definitely has an effect.

Acupuncture has become quite common in the UK over the last few years. So there's bound to be a good practitioner near you.

Cold Turkey

This is the most common method I know of. It doesn't cost anything and it's the route I chose. All you do is stop.

On the day in question, I woke up with a fairly substantial hangover and a mouth that felt like I'd been gargling bricks. (I'd been to some awards do or other the night before and like a lot of people, the more I drank the more I smoked).

I picked up my cigarettes for my morning fix with my coffee, and as I habitually went to light up, I realised that a cigarette was the last thing I felt like. So I put it back in the packet.

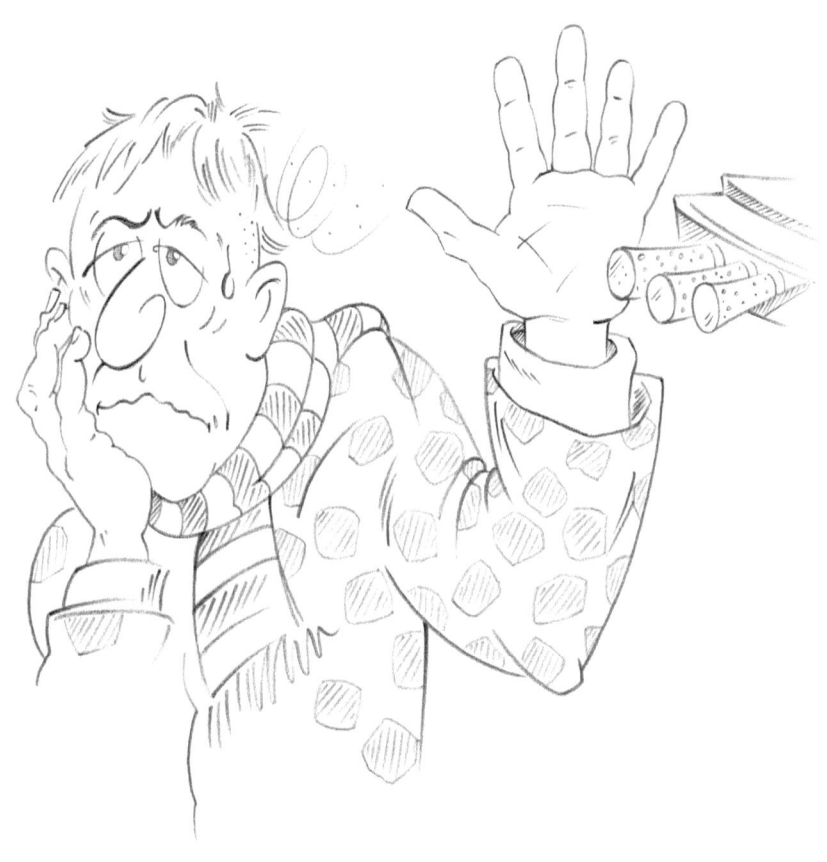

*A hangover or a touch of flu could
be an opportunity to stop*

A couple of hours went by and I still wasn't exactly gagging for a smoke. At this point a thought quietly occurred to me. Maybe as I wasn't in the mood for cigarettes, today was a good day to think about quitting.

I didn't commit myself to anything, I just thought I'd see if I could make it to lunch time without any nicotine.

Lunchtime came and went and I was still clean. So I thought, having got this far, I might as well go for it.

At which stage I realised I was committing myself to actually trying to stop.

So hangovers do have their uses.

Of course, I had withdrawal symptoms (the hangover just happened to be worse). And you can expect to get them, too.

And you'll notice that friends suddenly develop really aggravating habits, like reminding you about cigarettes at the very moment you've eventually succeeded in forgetting the damn things. You know the sort of thing; asking you how the non-smoking's going or complimenting you on your iron will, or even offering you a cigarette.

Then when you quite naturally snap at them, they smile knowingly and say stuff like, "giving up makes people bad tempered doesn't it".

Cold turkey isn't actually that hard and the withdrawal symptoms are mostly in your imagination.

Chemically, your dependence is over and done with in a couple of days.

As I'd found, many times before, the tough thing to shake in the long run, is the mental addiction.

Nicotine gum or patches:

You can get your nicotine fix without lighting up by using gum or patches. The idea is to reduce your withdrawal symptoms so your resolve doesn't weaken.

And while you're still getting nasty nicotine, at least your lungs are getting a break.

Patches don't do anything to break your addiction to nicotine though, and at some stage, you will have to deal with that.

Again if it works for you, go for it. But take care that you're not just putting off the dreaded day when you have to deal with it for good.

The slow cutdown:

Every smoker I've ever known has tried to cut down the number of cigarettes they smoke.

Plenty of them switched to low tar brands, too (although an old Health Education ad did rather aptly point out that switching to low tar is like jumping from the 17th floor instead of the 25th).

But obviously low tar is less harmful than high tar and ten a day is not as bad for you as 20. However I've never met anyone who actually managed to stop this way.

But again, if it works for you, it's right for you.

Hypnotism:

This works for some people, while others tell you all about their course of treatment at the same time as they light up.

If it works for you, great. If it doesn't, maybe you're looking for an easy way to do something which actually takes a bit of an effort. The important thing is not to give up giving up. Cigarettes are expensive and as you know, can cost you a lot more than money.

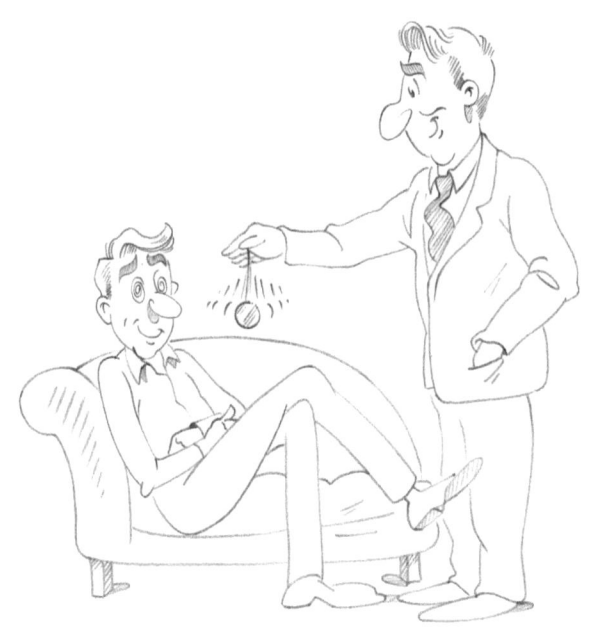

When you wake up you will no longer be a smoker

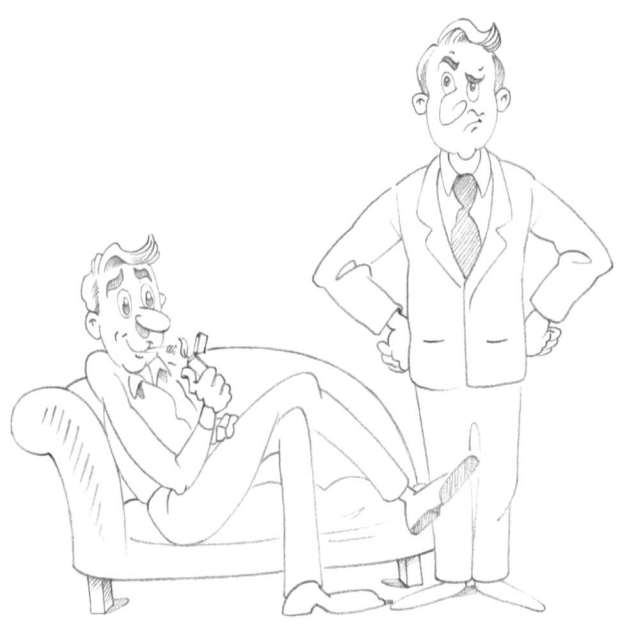

So how long does hypnotism take to work then?

There are dozens of ways that people approach this. The "how" doesn't matter, though. What really matters is that you do; "do" it, that is.

For some people searching for a way to stop is actually a trick they play on themselves in order to keep the habit going.

By endlessly searching for a way to stop that will really work for them, they can convince themselves they are "trying" to do what they need to do. But they somehow never quite find the right method. This means that in a twisted kind of way they contrive to give themselves permission to carry on smoking.

The truth is, you are the only one who can stop yourself smoking.

And actually, it's not that hard. If you don't think you can go without cigarettes for a whole day, just think about this; as I pointed out earlier, every night when you sleep, you stop smoking and go without any nicotine fixes for eight hours, maybe longer.

The chemical hold of nicotine isn't so strong.

The stopping part is OK, it's a little uncomfortable, but be in no doubt whatsoever - you can do it. And you have to get over that hurdle first before you do the bit that's really important.

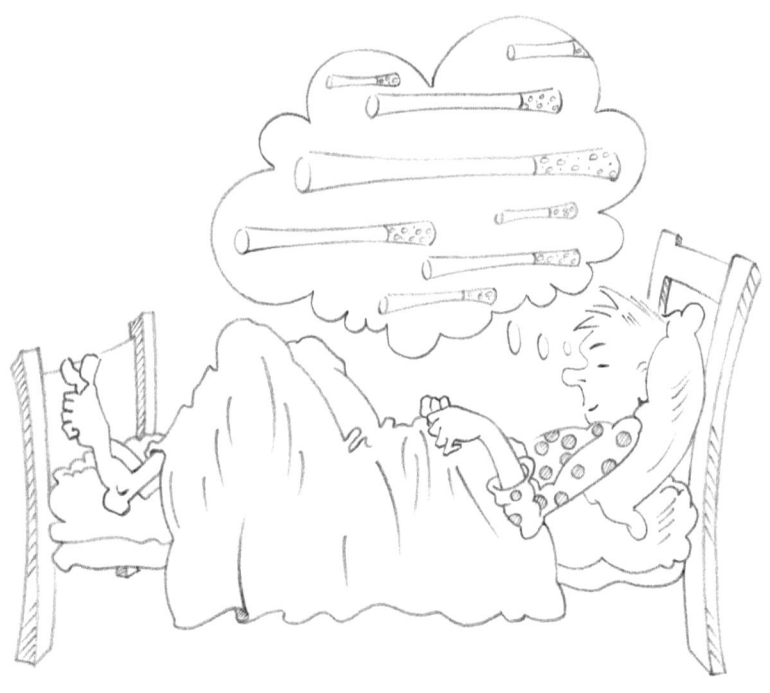

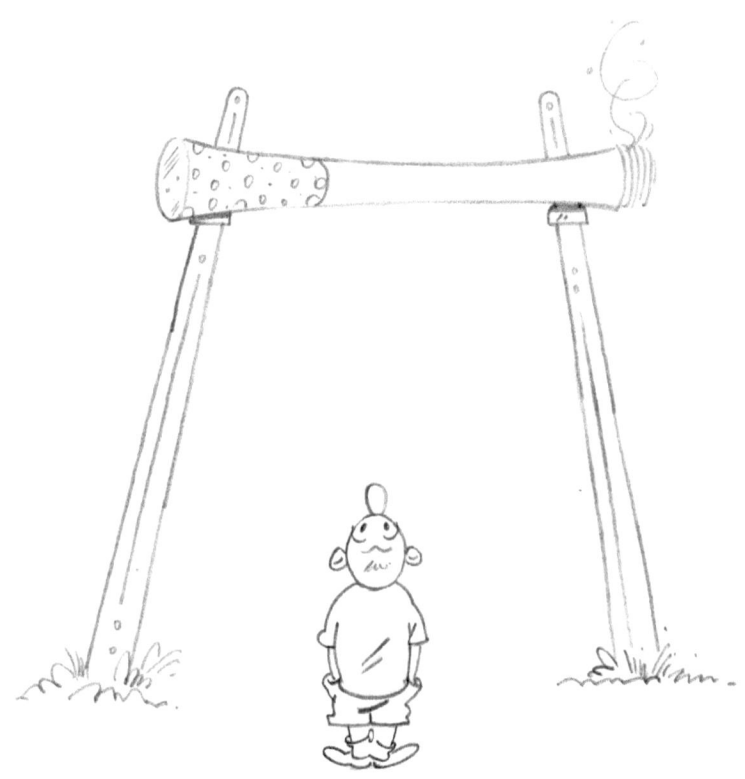

You can get over it

Becoming a non smoker.

A non smoker is not someone, like a recovering alcoholic, who manages their addiction so as not to give in to it again. A non smoker is someone who has no need to smoke nor any desire to do so.

By following the techniques described in this guide, I became a genuine non smoker. I did it in a remarkably short time and with very little effort.

And if I (someone who sometimes used to smoke three packs of American High Tar cigarettes every day) can do it, you can too.

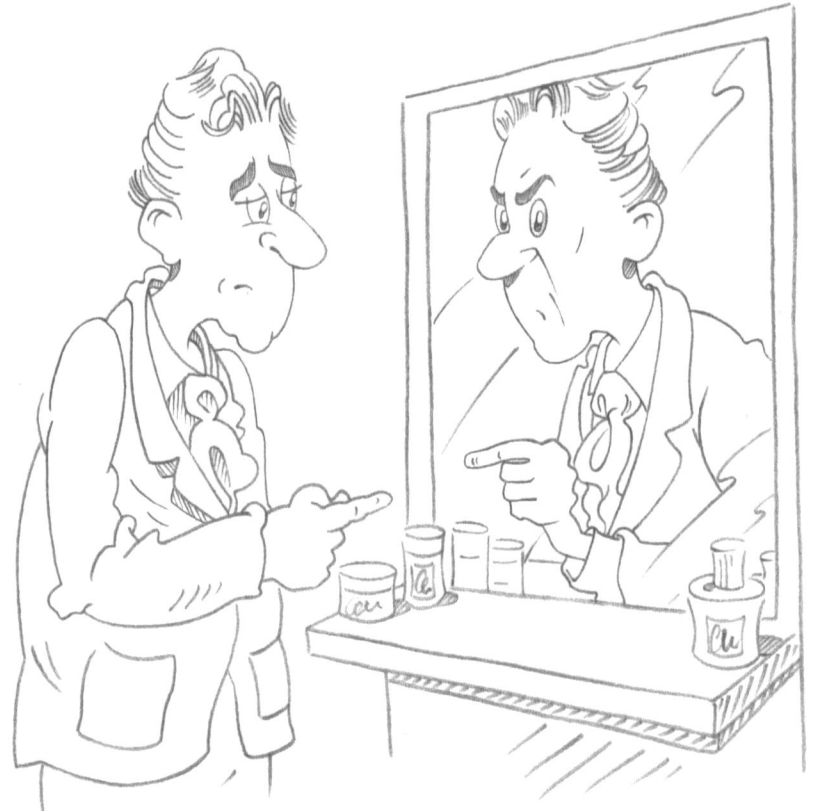

Step 3. Take action

Don't just stop. Start.

If you think about it, even the language associated with breaking the nicotine habit, makes it harder. It's all negative.

According to what people say, you don't "start" being healthier, improving your circulation, smelling more pleasant and breathing cleaner air, you "stop" smoking. You don't "take up" clean lungs, unclogged arteries and the ability to taste food, you "give up" cigarettes. It's the language of self deprivation and by using it, every time you think about breaking the nicotine habit (50 times a day probably to start with), you make yourself feel you're being deprived of something

The classic reaction to this, is to redouble the resolve, reinforce the will power and resist the urge as hard as possible. Which makes it harder. Because resisting temptation is passive. It's also negative - you are trying to make yourself "not" do something. For ever.

And every time you think of, or want cigarettes, it makes you feel like you're being weak which makes you feel bad about yourself so you try even harder to resist. This negative cycle reinforces itself. Because a part of your mind keeps telling you that anything you have to resist with this much effort, must be pretty special.

So the harder you resist, the harder you have to resist. No wonder so many people who stop, end up starting again.

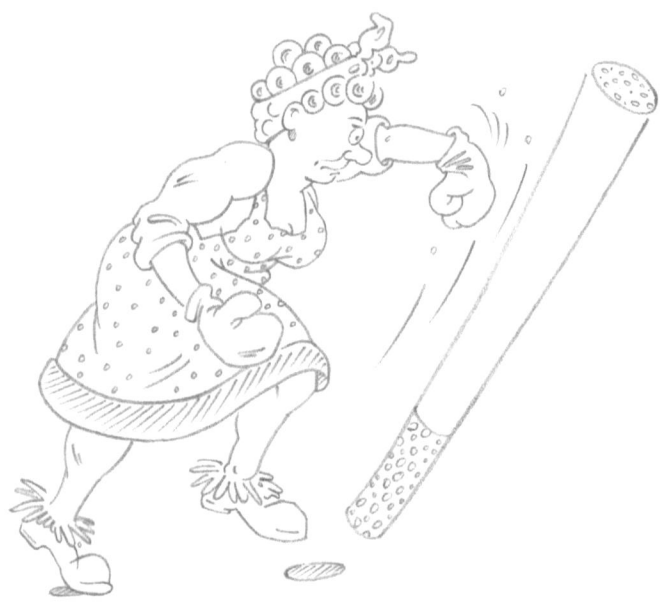

You can beat it

This occurred to me when, just before I broke the habit for good myself, I spoke to a friend who'd not smoked for two or three years. I suggested that after all this time, he must have completely broken the habit. He laughed (a little maniacally, actually) and told me not a day went by when he didn't crave for a cigarette.

What he said stayed with me and when I eventually made the break, I thought, "what if, instead of giving up smoking, I took up non smoking, freed myself from the nicotine prison, did my lungs a favour, improved my cardio vascular system, saved myself thousands of pounds, got my sense of taste and smell back.. etc? Would that help me to break the hold that nicotine always had on me in the past.?"

The answer is a resounding, positive "yes"

Once I started looking at it this way, I suddenly found that, instead of resisting the irresistible, I felt I had a weapon to use against the habit and instead of passively waiting for it to go away I could actively do something to make it go away.

My frame of mind became increasingly more positive. Simply looking at things this way every time I felt the urge to smoke, gave me a weapon against the habit.

It gave me a way to get satisfaction from beating nicotine. In fact, I even started to enjoy encounters between nicotine desire and me because I knew at last that instead of burying it in my unconscious and hoping it wouldn't nag me too much, I could actually beat it. I could win.

So if you want to stay stopped, get your mind set right. Be positive about what you're doing. You're not giving up, you're starting something. You're beating nicotine. You're getting clean. You're getting fitter. You're cutting your chances of lung cancer, You're avoiding heart disease and dozens of other nasty things. You're breathing clean air.

Don't just stay with the positives I used. Invent your own. Make them personal. Make them funny. The important thing is to take charge of it. Once you do that, you're well on your way.

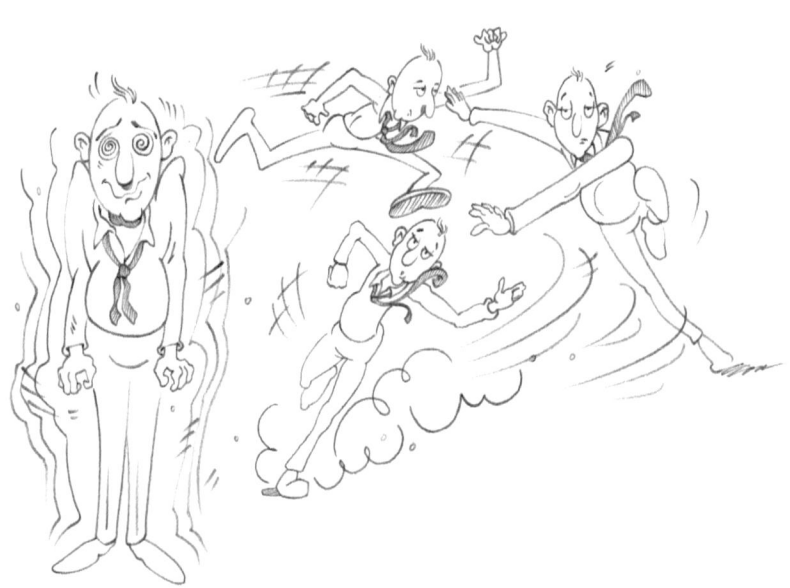

You'll have a lot more energy

Step 4. Make it work for you

Energy Bursts

Something that struck me in the first few days after I broke my habit, was how the craving for a cigarette seemed to express itself as restless, negative energy. I would find myself fidgeting, standing up, sitting down, glancing around to check things I'd checked just a few seconds before and so on.

This restlessness was a kind of raw energy that didn't seem to have anywhere to go. And it could feel pretty uncomfortable. The more I tried to ignore it or make it go away, the more it nagged at me.

I realised this was exactly how it felt when I "needed" a cigarette while I was addicted. The difference was, then I made the restlessness go away with a cigarette.

So by fighting these bad energy rushes, I was actually building up a craving in my mind. And as usual, making things harder for myself.

Then I had an idea. I thought, what if, instead of fighting these restless energy bursts, I harnessed them and actually put them to work for me? Wouldn't that be a pretty positive way of fighting?

The next time I felt this rush of energy, I used it to work out what positive things I could use energy bursts for. I sat down and wrote a list of all the things I wanted to achieve. Big things, small things, personal things, political things... they all went in.

Before I'd even got the first item on the list, the negative craving had gone. I wrote lots of lists after that. My first one looked something like this:

- make appointment for eye test
- talk to job agency about getting a better job
- prune roses
- go for run
- call friends - make list of friends I haven't spoken to for a while
- fill in tax return.

Then every time I felt that rush of bad energy, I did something from the list. When the list was used up, I wrote a new one and worked my way through that.

By about list number three, my lists were getting quite ambitious and I was including things on them like writing a book to help other people kick the nicotine habit. This is it. Not exactly a book, more a booklet. But a lot more satisfying and far more useful than a cigarette.

Before long, I actually started to enjoy the energy rushes, even to look forward to them. I started to associate them with getting things done. And before long, the association with cigarettes simply melted away. So instead of lighting up next time you feel the craving, do something for yourself.

Making use of energy rushes like this is a way of actively attacking your smoking habit and it helps you to start making the transition from someone who wants a cigarette but can't have one, to someone who simply doesn't want one and in fact has better things to do than smoke.

More generally, it's also a way of dropping habits you don't like and replacing them with things that are of real use to you. You don't just have to apply it to smoking, you can apply it to all parts of your life. Who knows what you'll achieve if you do.

- -

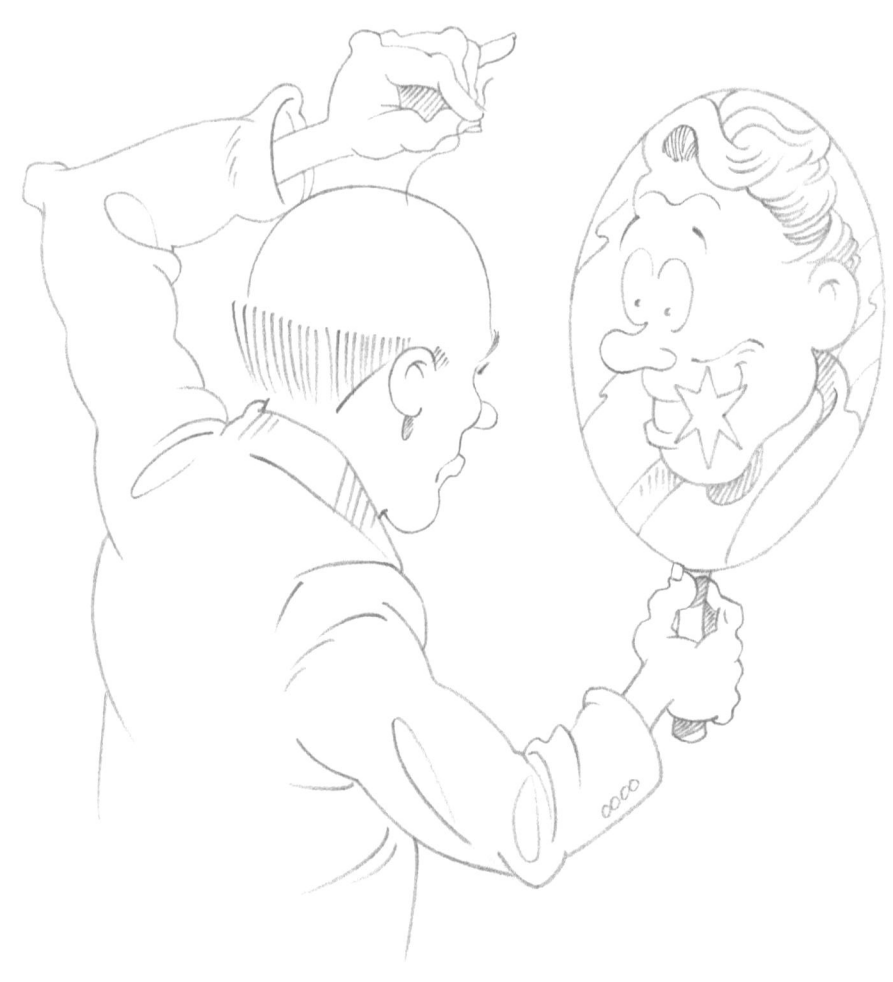

Picture yourself the way you'd like to be

Step 5. Picture it

Seeing yourself as a non smoker is one step from being one. One of the tricks addiction plays on the mind is to sneak into your unconscious and associate itself with your personality.

Cigarettes become part of your routine, part of the little habits and mannerisms that separate you as an individual from other people.

In this way, they con you into thinking they are part of who you are.

We are all addicted to being who we are. And when you close down the nicotine habit, you unconsciously feel like you are closing down parts of yourself:

- The person who started each day with a coffee and a cigarette, was you.
- The person who always smoked a luxurious cigarette after sex, was you.
- The person who enjoyed a drink and a conversation over a king size, was you.
- The person who lit up a King size when things got a bit stressed, was you.
- The person who enjoyed the Sunday papers over a filter tip, was you.
- The person who did practically anything with a lit cigarette on the go, was you.

Add them up. You'll be amazed how many parts of your life have an association with cigarettes. You may have not thought about it consciously, but unconsciously at least, part of your mind will have been totting up just how many parts of your previous behaviour (which feels like your very personality) will have to go. And that part of your mind doesn't like change. It's got used to you being you and wants to keep things as they are. So it will instantly start putting obstacles in your way and making things feel as difficult as possible.

In order to really break the hold of nicotine, you have to deal with this aspect of the problem. If you don't, then every time you pick up a coffee, drink a glass of wine, answer the phone, go into a pub or do any of the dozens of little things you do every day, part of you will nag and fret, wondering why there isn't a cigarette attached.

Dealing with it though, is so easy and simple, you probably won't believe it. Not 'til you try it that is.

First, it's worth checking your mindset. Remind yourself to be positive. You're not depriving yourself, not giving up anything. What you're doing is beating nicotine, becoming someone who doesn't smoke and doesn't want to.

Next, write a list. (I told you there were a lot of lists). You could use your next nicotine energy burst to do this. The list should contain all the tiny bits of habitual behaviour and mannerisms you associate with the habit and all the things you use cigarettes for.

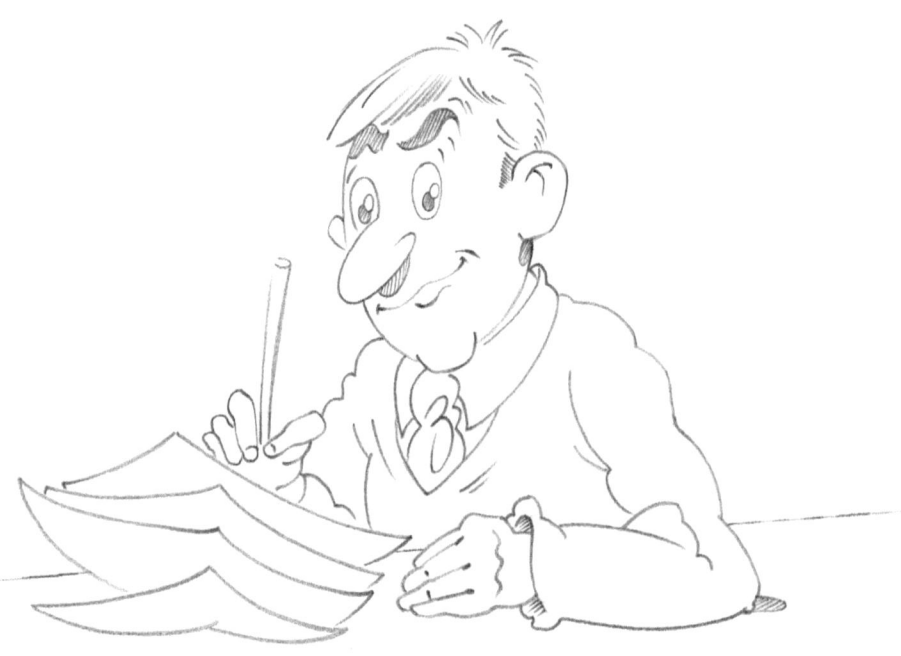

I'm writing a list of all the reasons why I hate writing lists

The part of your mind that resists change will find it harder to resist when you do this because these associated habits are almost always trivial. So when you consciously set them out in front of yourself and look at them, they really don't seem very important. Certainly not important enough to be worth the risk of cancer, heart disease, blindness etc etc.

I found the best way to make sure the list was comprehensive was to divide it into three headed sections:

----

1. Things I do when I smoke

This includes things like, how you light a cigarette - do you use matches or a lighter? How do you hold the cigarette? Which hand? Are you a deep inhaler? Do you like to blow smoke rings? Do you smoke the whole cigarette? Do you normally carry your cigarettes in the left or right pocket? Or do you carry them in a bag? Do you use cigarettes as an excuse to stop for a moment? Do you use cigarettes as a spur to action?

The important thing is to look at your own habits and draw as comprehensive a picture as you can of them. Especially the really trivial ones.

2. Times and places I like to smoke

Do you smoke when you drive? In bed? Out in the fresh air?

After breakfast? After dinner? Over coffee? On the phone? On holiday? Over a drink? After exercise? In the pub? Over a crossword? Last thing at night? First thing in the morning? Remember, this isn't an either/or list. Every little detail of your habit goes in.

----

3. Things I use smoking for

Do you smoke to calm yourself down when you get nervous? To wake yourself up? To look cool? To help you concentrate? To help you relax? As an ice breaker with new people? To create a momentary pause while you think? To avoid doing things?

It doesn't matter whether you complete this three part list straight away. What's important is to start getting it down - you can always add things later as they occur to you. To begin with, you probably won't realise just how insidiously the habit has wrapped itself round your life, anyway.

The nicotine habit is a bit like a computer virus, or one of those irritating bits of software you want to chuck off your PC but when you get rid of the application folder you find there are dozens of associated files hidden all over your hard disk.

Fortunately, you're not a computer and your knowledge of yourself is better than anyone else's. So you don't need an I.T. Man to unpick this nasty bug. You are the best person for the job. That's why it's important to be honest and to get even your most trivial smoking habits down on paper.

When you've made your list, go through it and put a mark by anything you think you'll find it really difficult to do without. Also mark anything you see as important to your personality.

You'll be surprised by how few you mark. For me, there were only two of any significance.

First; like many writers, I used smoking as part of my work habit. Picking up a pencil was synonymous with lighting a cigarette. So my big fear was that when I stopped smoking, I wouldn't be able to write any more.

Second; I used smoking to keep my appetite under control. So I worried that without the cigarettes I'd get fat. Simply writing these things down and owning up to them, helps deal with them. Get the enemy out in plain view and it's suddenly much clearer what you have to do to beat him.

The next thing to do is to mentally clear smoker and smoking associations from your mind and start building a nicotine-free self image for yourself.

The New You

The image you have of yourself is as a smoker. Even after you stop. So many things you do, and have done, in your life will throw up smoking associations.

I found the following easy and deceptively simple exercise, incredibly helpful. It only takes a few moments and you can do it practically anywhere, any time.

First, look at the list you just made and choose one thing off it. It doesn't matter which. The trivial stuff is just as important as the big issues, maybe more important.

Sit quietly somewhere and relax. Close your eyes, take a deep breath then exhale slowly.

Now, picture yourself doing what you chose from your list (driving the car, enjoying a glass of wine drinking coffee, reading a novel, whatever... it doesn't matter which). Picture it in every detail, notice how well you are doing it. Notice how enjoyable the experience is.

Notice you are not smoking.

That's it. You have already started to repair your self image. It's so simple you may find it hard to believe, but it really is a powerful way to change things and it really does work.

Over the next few days and energy bursts, work your way through your lists until you have "seen" every aspect of your smoking self in a non smoking light. And seen yourself as a non smoker in every situation you can imagine. Then start at the beginning and work your way through the list again.

It's important to "see" yourself as a non smoker, rather than just telling yourself you're one. Seeing really is believing.

It's also important to be as positive as possible. Don't conjure up negative, boring or self deprecating images of yourself. In this case, flattery really will get you everywhere. Admire yourself and have all the other people in your image, admire you and your actions, too.

Remember these are your images. If you can't star in your own images, what can you star in?

If you have a secret fear, or reservation, that your mind keeps using to block your efforts (mine was not being able to write without cigarettes), simply visualise yourself as not having the fear. It will soon fade.

This visualisation exercise may sound too simple and too easy, but it really is effective. And if you feel a bit daft doing it, just remember you used to stick a rolled up piece of paper filled with dried weeds, in your mouth, then light it and inhale all kinds of noxious, foul smelling stuff into your lungs. If that's not daft, I don't know what is. So if you used to do that, let's face it you don't really mind looking daft, do you?

Earlier in this booklet, I made a list of the reasons why smoking isn't worth doing and suggested you did the same. Now for a more positive list.

For the record, here are few reasons why it IS worth being a non smoker. Read the list, then make one of your own, adding any reasons you think are good and using any parts of mine that are particularly pertinent to you.

Being a NON SMOKER is good because:

- It's healthy
- My breath doesn't smell
- My clothes don't smell
- I don't turn other people into passive smokers
- Now I can be smug and feel superior to people who do smoke
- I like myself as a non smoker
- I save money
- I can taste and smell things again
- I'm fitter
- I'm not setting a bad example to children
- I'm not clogging up my arteries
- I don't cough all the time
- My risk of heart disease and lung cancer is less
- My brain is getting more oxygen
- Life insurance is cheaper
- I'm not giving money to cynical nicotine peddlers (aka tobacco companies)

People worry that all sorts of things will happen when they kick the habit - two that seem to come up a lot are:

1 They'll put on weight.

2 They'll be nervous wrecks.

All that's happening here is the part of the mind that doesn't like change is putting up a bit of a fight. Simply deciding to treat food cravings or feelings of tension as energy bursts, will help.

So will visualising yourself as a non smoker who doesn't suffer from whatever problem it is. But you can do more.

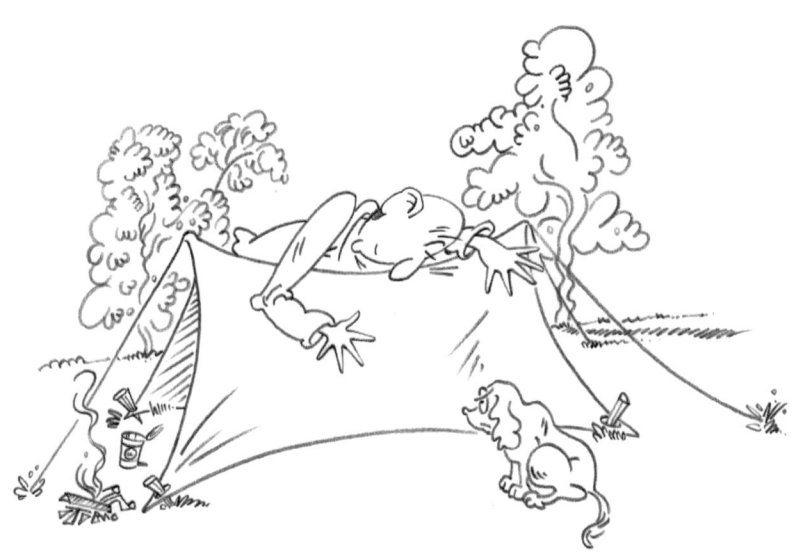

You may start feeling tents

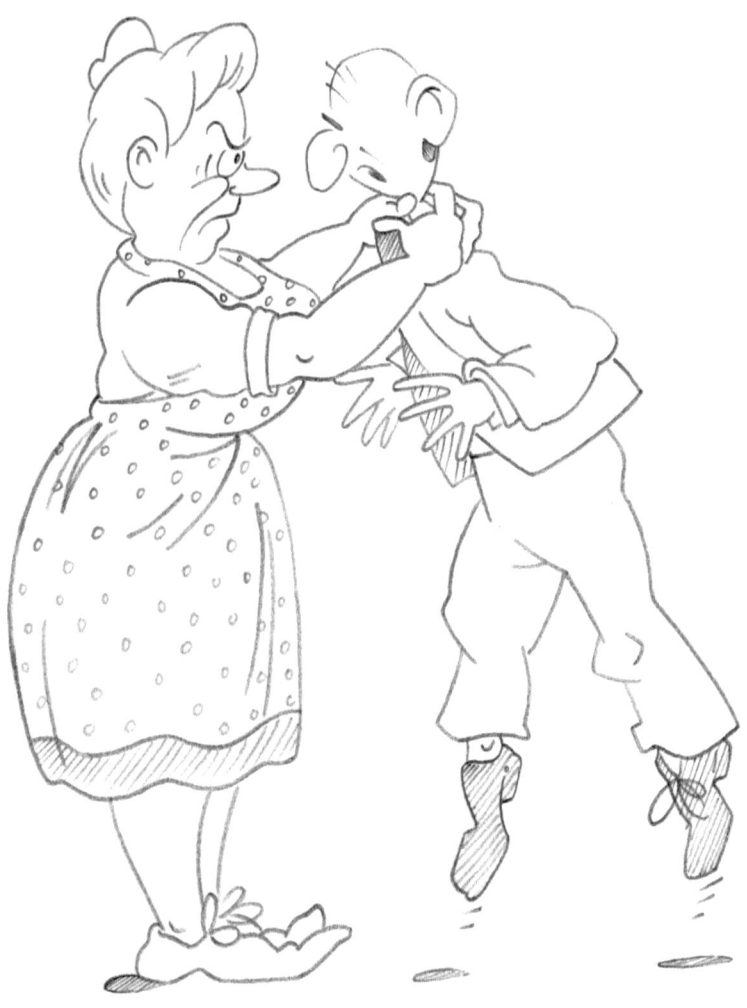

There are many ways to relieve tension

Food cravings:

If you decide to treat food cravings as energy bursts, you could use these bursts to do something which fundamentally undermines your fears. If you did two press ups or touched your toes twice, every time you felt a food craving, you'd probably be in better shape in a week than you ever were in years as a smoker.

By burning energy, you'd also be earning yourself the right to more food, in the process.

If you want a slight change to routine, use some of the energy bursts to stop for a moment and visualise yourself as a slim, fit, healthy person. Notice that you don't have a cigarette and don't feel like one either.

Another thing you can do is to make sure you have plenty of the kinds of food around that fill you up but don't make you fat.

So even if you make food cravings go away with food, they won't make you fat. Stock up with fruit, celery, raw carrots, high fibre stuff

The intensity of the food cravings dies down quite quickly. What's important is not to get into the habit of eating the wrong sorts of things as snacks.

It shouldn't be long before your appetite settles down from voracious to healthy. And if you have made a habit of snacking on good stuff, you shouldn't really put on weight.

Six months after I stopped smoking, my weight was down by 3lbs "Smug git", you may think, but the point is, if I who can't walk past a tub of ice cream without inhaling the entire contents, can stop smoking and not turn into a house on legs, you can too.

Tension

At some time or other, most smokers use cigarettes as pacifiers. To calm down after a shock, to settle themselves when they feel nervous, to regain their equilibrium after anger or fear etc. For some people, nicotine is almost a tranquilliser. So while you're kicking the habit, you're bound to feel tense from time to time. In fact, it would be really surprising if you didn't.

The first thing to do is to simply accept the feelings as a natural reaction to kicking nicotine. And next time you feel on edge, to see the tension as an energy burst. Then, it may sound contradictory, but you can now use the energy to relax.

There are loads of relaxation techniques. From meditation to polishing the family silver to digging the garden. Doesn't matter which one you plump for, so long as it works for you.

Here's one you can try.

Sit back in your chair. Take a deep breath then exhale slowly. Close your eyes. Concentrate on your breathing, inhaling and exhaling slowly.

Now working upwards from your feet, think about each part of your body, one piece at a time.

Imagine your feet becoming heavier and heavier, all by themselves. Then your legs. Then your hands and arms. And so on, 'til every part of you feels like it is sinking into the chair.

Feel your shoulders becoming loose, feel the tension leaving your neck. Now, still breathing slowly, give all the tension you have ever felt an imagined physical form. See it as something breakable or disposable. Maybe it's a tightly wound spring in a clock or a kettle, or a stretched rubber band or maybe if you prefer, it's just an ugly, nasty, sharp spiky thing.

Now imagine your tension being destroyed by whatever method pleases you the most. Drop the clock with its tightly wound spring from the top floor of the highest building you know. Watch it shatter into pieces on the ground. Or blow the spiky thing to smithereens. Whatever image gives you the most pleasure.

Another relaxation technique is the parachute.

Close your eyes, take a deep breath and exhale slowly. Now imagine you're very high up and floating under an enormous parachute.

Your altimeter reads 10 thousand feet.

Imagine that there are ten "strengths" of the tension you feel. You are currently at maximum - Force 10. As you descend on the parachute, you will reach lower tension "strengths". Down to force nine at 9,000 feet, force 8 at 8,000 feet and so on.

Allow yourself 5 seconds to get to 9 thousand feet, counting yourself down slowly 5, 4, 3, 2, 1 and noticing how each second you count you are just a little more relaxed.

Pause at each level for a few moments to appreciate the lessening tension, before counting yourself down to 8,000 feet. Then gradually work your way down to ground level like this, where you will feel absolutely peaceful and calm.

Enjoy the feeling of relaxed calm for as long as you like before carrying on with whatever you were doing before.

Another way to release tension is exercise. You might try chopping logs or hitting a punch bag - two very satisfying ways of transferring anger onto something inanimate while getting the old heart and lungs working, too.

If you can't find something you can hit without getting arrested, try just pushing a wall as hard as you can for a few seconds. You'll be surprised how much better you feel (make sure it's a strong wall though).

If the tension is rising to screaming pitch, try going somewhere you won't be overheard and just scream the place down. It might give you a sore throat, but it certainly gets rid of tension.

Finally, a useful release mechanism that takes just a few moments is this. Take a deep breath and hold it. Now tense up every muscle you've got, tighter and tighter and tighter until you feel like you're going to burst. Hold onto this for as long as you can, then let everything go floppy at once and let your breath explode out. Repeat as often as necessary.

These tension release exercises are really useful. They won't just help you deal with the stress of nicotine withdrawal, they will help you deal with tension and stress wherever and whenever it crops up in your life.

And finally

Well, there you are that's it. Or at least, that's it, apart from this last bit.

What I've tried to do is to write a simple and easy guide that will help you become a genuine non smoker. Someone who doesn't need or want nicotine and doesn't need to avoid other smokers or smoking situations. Someone for whom the cigarette habit is completely gone from their life. As opposed to someone who is desperate for a ciggy but fighting the desire with every ounce of will power they can muster

If you have your doubts about the methods, tricks and ideas I'm suggesting here and you're still in that doubt zone between giving up and lighting up, all I can say is it worked for me. And not only did it work, but once I hit on this approach, it was actually very easy.

I'm not one of those annoying health fascists who's never smoked but still feels qualified to tell you how to stop. I used to smoke - a lot. And I did so for about 15 years. So I understand what a tough ride it can be and the very real problems that can go with it.

Which means that if I say it's possible to beat nicotine and that you can beat it with very little effort and that you can basically, erase the habit from your life for good, you know there's at least a possibility you can.

This guide is a tool kit you can use to actively DO something to fight nicotine, rather than passively trying to avoid it. It will help you identify the enemy in all its subtle guises and work out strategies and tactics to outwit it. And to beat it.

If you follow my suggestions, the process of becoming a non smoker can be relatively smooth and free of strife.

But don't feel you have to religiously follow everything I say. In fact, the process might even work better if you adapt my suggestions to suit your own personality and include your own ideas. The important thing is that you realise nicotine is not bigger than you. Don't let it bully you. You can beat it.

However, I can't make you do it. The only person that can beat nicotine for you, is you.

- -

www.ingramcontent.com/pod-product-compliance
Ingram Content Group UK Ltd.
Pitfield, Milton Keynes, MK11 3LW, UK
UKHW041433180426
11947UKWH00007B/424